FLOWERS FROM MY QUIET STORM

A Mental Health Narrative from A Family's Perspective

FLOWERS FROM MY QUIET STORM

A Mental Health Narrative from A Family's Perspective

Chaplain Delora Ann

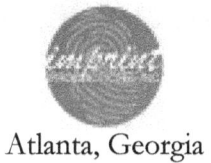

Atlanta, Georgia

Flowers From My Quiet Storm
A Mental Health Narrative from A Family's Perspective

© 2021 Chaplain Delora Ann

All rights reserved. No part of this publication may be reproduced or transmitted in any form or by any means without the written permission of the publisher.

ISBN 978-1-7358124-7-2

All services completed by Imprint Productions Inc. Printed in the United States of America
Published by Imprint Production Inc. info@imprintproductionsinc.com

Self-Help Memoirs
First Edition 2021

10 9 8 7 6 5 4 3 2 1

CONTENTS

Author's Note	1
Preface: Mental Illness the Face of Conflict	3
Dedication	5
Acknowledgments	6
Introduction	14
Statement of Support	22
Reflections	23
Chapter 1: Clueless	28
Chapter 2: Caught off Guard	35
Chapter 3: A Vicious Cycle of Mental Illness	43
Chapter 4: Blindsided	51
Self-Care	59
Afterword	62
Resources	65

AUTHOR'S NOTE

WORRY ABOUT WHAT OTHER PEOPLE THINK (NAMI-Family Perspective)

People who suffer with mental illness have to hold themselves to some accountability. Although I worried about what other people thought, I didn't mean we should put up with the hostility, bad language(profanity), and insults from the sufferer with this disease. This Behavior can break us at a point if we don't be proactive and push back in a positive way, of course. "Les Brown," I quote, "it will stay in your face until you deal with it with Grace, you can't make this stuff up". This statement sums it up for me. I will share with you the real-life situations of a family who has been tried in the fire, so to speak (1 Peter 1:7). We thank God for His Grace and for teaching us how to respond to others that are mentally sick. After all that's said and done, we have to LOVE them in, and when you've done all you can with housing them, praying for them, and giving them resources that some, not all of them reject, there isn't much else left to do except let them go on with the lives God gave them.

My cousin, Connie Harper, and I had a conversation about mental illness in our family. She shared with me her major challenge in the past, which was not having anyone to help. She stated that there was always conflict, but after the conflict, those with this illness always come back with an improved response.

This seems contradictory, but it works because I've witnessed recovery from individuals that are writing books, Working jobs, holding speaking engagements, and enlightening the world that they, people with diagnoses, do recover. Why? Because to be delivered and set free, I believe one has to accept their illness. God has forgiven them as well, the sufferer has to forgive those who have hurt them and be free from bitterness in forgiveness, which is tough. Taking the proper medication is hard for them, too. Because of HIPPA Laws, the individual has his or their own rights to do whatever they deem is best for them and their life.

I didn't always know how to articulate this way of life God gave me in the mental health ministry. I care about helping those in need because whether it would be a movement, women's church ministry, or a cause, it comes naturally for me. I want to be there to support and help in serving other families who are just like us. My goal is to continue with this mandate for the rest of my earthly life as God wills, ensuring we get the message of hope to the community.

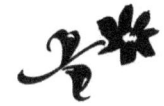

PREFACE

Mental Illness the Face of Conflict

Now over 40 years later, mental illness shows up at my doorstep; This is something I didn't raise my hand for, and since being catapulted into it, I have to learn to accept it. Inconveniences are sometimes necessary. I heard the Holy Spirit say to me at 4 am one morning, this book and some illustrations are real stories of a parent's obstacles with loved ones stricken with mental illness and their ability to cope. We don't name diagnoses because they are not their illness but have a disease that causes them in their human condition to have day-to-day struggles in their lives. Over the years, I developed parts of this book, putting thoughts on paper to make this become a reality for us as a whole, with the intention to help others just as my supporters helped my family and me.

We have been in COVID-19 PANDEMIC since 2019; now, halfway through the year into 2021, we are still pressing through. I realize the truth has to be told to help break the stigma. While listening to the news media, along with watching cases rise in families and the communities at large, Mental illness in every way has become the face of conflict. Because of these unprecedented times and changes, sharing a family's perspective I truly believe is God's timing. The objective, prayer, goal, and desire in writing these memoirs are to give a better understanding and dispel negative comments and reactions from others less empathetic.

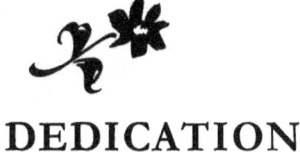

DEDICATION

This book is dedicated to our four very strong, determined, loving, and amazing adult children and our little grandchildren.

They have a very special place in society, in our hearts, and we pray our real-life experiences will help other families. As a family, we have been vigilant in overcoming stigma through recovery, attending support groups and networking with the mental health movement for several years. The fact that three of our adult children clinically diagnosed and one denied diagnosis from a college counselor has led me to share openly with readers our trials and tribulations. We all need to be free from feeling the shame, guilt, and frustration this illness brings with it. For if the Son has set us free, we will be free indeed. (John 8:36)

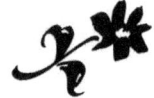

ACKNOWLEDGMENTS

All the Glory belongs to You, O God, for setting this platform and sending me the support to write these memoirs, I'd love to acknowledge all my supporters, but I would be remiss if I didn't mention a few of them and pray; I haven't overlooked anyone. A very special thanks to them all.

A huge thanks to my marketing team NueWay, Imprint Productions, Inc. It's not easy finding the right fit to help your dream or vision become a reality.

I'll first mention Ashley Smith', author, mother, entrepreneur. writing coach, peer mentor, state trainer for NAMI (National Alliance on Mental Illness) movement, IOOV (IN OUR OWN VOICE) presenter. Recently, we reconnected by divine intervention after losing contact for a few years. Our 2nd daughter and Ashley became very good friends and colleagues. Our daughter reached out to her on a Thursday in crisis- Ashley, assisted my daughter, Ashley and her family as best as she could. She offered them room and board overnight. Little did I know that Ashley had a need which was to drive to Sacramento, California to visit her 9-year-old son she affectionately calls "Big Boy " and her family. By Monday, we were on a road trip by car crossing seven-state lines. I will never be the same after this experience. It has humbled me. Ashley is a loving mommy and author of two books with two more under way. She is a beacon of light in the mental health community and the world. I truly adore her and her family and really appreciate her support for my family and me during these very difficult times.

One day I asked Missionary/Minister Marjory Patrick, author, wife, mother, and grandmother, church member and ministry leader of Global Missions for her input. I believe the Lord appointed her mentorship to me. She gave me the most beautiful words of encouragement, and I quote," Beloved of the Lord, Delora remember:

1. One word at a time equals a sentence
2. One sentence at a time equals a paragraph
3. One paragraph at a time equals a page
4. One page at a time equals a chapter
5. One chapter at a time equals a book!

These words help propel me forward.
Trust God's timing.

I would be remiss not to mention several of the NAMI members by name including: Pat Strode, NAMI Movement mommy/advocate works at the Georgia Public Safety Training Center along with CIT (Crisis Intervention Team). During her tenure with NAMI as an employee, she made a huge impact among medical professionals, families, and the mental health community while dealing with her own family members with mental health challenges. Continuing to work behind the scenes, she's responsible for getting me involved with the NAMI Movement years ago.

Chaplain Annette is a military wife and veteran herself, and is also a part of the NAMI movement. Their story, like hundreds of other families, is all too familiar. One day I answered a phone call referral from the NAMI Office helpline. As Annette began to express her issues about her loved one with a diagnosis, I listened tentatively. I believe the Lord moved by His spirit, connected the both of us. As she opened up about her faith in God and the strength she gained through trusting Him, she was led to recruit me into the chaplaincy program of studies. When I asked her how she accomplished these strides with her present challenges, her reply was, spending time under her mentorship. To God Be All the Glory!

Vikki Holloway, NAMI facilitator, along with her mother, Josephine Chappell, held meetings at Auburn Family Support Group, which later merged to become Atlanta/Auburn Family Support Group. Encouraged by the late Don and Jean Dervan told me how to connect with and create a merger for the Atlanta/Auburn Group because there wasn't one for the Metro area, so we did. Vikki shared a phrase that she created in the form of a question, "If my brain is sick, would you bring me flowers"? What a remarkable way to acknowledge those who suffer with mental illness because it's not embraced readily the way cancer, diabetes, or other medical conditions. One day she convinced me to step up because she was ready to take a back seat from facilitating, and I accepted.

Keith Lee, a NAMI facilitator family member, and Military Veteran, led meetings at the Helene Mills Senior Facility. His loved one suf- fered from mental illness giving him the opportunity to care for his granddaughter. His commitment to the NAMI Movement goes beyond reproach. Words of appreciation and encouragement are priceless in thanking him for all his hard work, dedication, leadership, and for holding those family support groups.

Iola Anyan, a NAMI Facilitator family member, led meetings at the Helene Mills Senior Facility. She still remains in our hearts for her commitment, love, and support. Iola shared information and resources like housing and support- ive employment that really helped her sibling before moving to the Washington of D.C.

Eric Ferguson, NAMI Connection Support Group Facilitator, moved from New York and called the NAMI office, who then forwarded my phone number to him. Passionate about supporting peers, we con- nected, and the work began with assisting him in getting a space to hold Connections Support meetings that continued for several years. His tireless efforts have not gone unnoticed.

Stephanie Tyree, NAMI IOOV Presenter, Art Instructor who vol- unteered her time at the local community center, she too is a product of the NAMI Movement and has created many art pieces, one of which I use and practice as a philosophy in my life that says:

"I Enjoy Serving Others and Know that Serving Others is what I'm Called To Do"

Beverly Phillips, Entrepreneur and NAMI Mommy along with their beloved son; the late Mr. Kenneth Phillips (Kenya's husband), and Kenya Dual Master Degree College Graduate in ministry, author, NAMI Georgia State Peer Trainer for IOOV, Grief & Recovery Coach helped Co-teach Family to Family a 12-week training class at Atlanta/Auburn Group, as We tagged team; teaching families how to overcome the daily challenges we all face.

Ms. Cindy Bohannon Brown, Professional Educator and NAMI Movement Member for mental illness, has helped support families and children, giving her financial support, time, and energy creating her own project, "HUGS For Humanity".

Chaplain Delora Ann

Kim Jones, Executive Director NAMI Georgia State office, and Mommy attended a training I participated in at the Fulton County Sheriff's Office. It was after hearing my presentation that she came up to me, gave me a huge hug expressing she didn't know my mental health story; Then she bought me lunch. I appreciate her empathy and kindness.

Faye Taylor, President of NAMI, Georgia Board Member and Mommy, wrote an awesome letter of recommendation when I asked if she could support me in a special endeavor. She also advocates for her family as well as supporting the community of families with mental health challenges.

Agent Trebor Randall of GBI and I met at former Agent Debbie Shaw's CIT class of the Georgia Public Safety Training Center. I also had the opportunity to participate with them both in a training session. Debbie coordi- nated, under the former Georgia Governor Deal. They put a mandate in place. The goal continues to train all law enforcers and other agencies that interact with the mental health community of families. His wife; Lady Deal, set in on a week's training, familiarizing herself with this process as well. Debbie also role-plays in de-escalation training tech- niques in the CIT class.

Major Charlene Heard, former Fulton County Sheriff's Office, Train to Trainer Instructor, former CIT Coordinator for Georgia Public Safety Training Center, set the tone in her passion for and commitment to our incarcerated mental health population and community of families while serving over 25 years of service. She participated in videos used as training modules of real-life experiences written by Police Officers, which she role played in for several years.

Major Chuck Simmons, former Henry County Police Department, now coordinates CIT for Georgia Public Safety Training Center, holding weekly training's and pulling together acting novices, getting them to role-play mental illness scenes portraying families in real-life crisis. He also role -plays de-escalation training techniques in the CIT class, working after retirement with our families and community.

Officer Cerrina Leeks Holt, former Atlanta Police Department Training Center facilitator now coordinator for Georgia Public Safety Training Center, CIT training class supporting our community of families with mental illness and has given me valuable resources in my time of need in crisis. This is not the first time she has been acknowledged for her committed work in the community.

Lieutenant Twantta Jennings, former Fulton County Sheriff's Office, Train to Trainer Instructor, now coordinates CIT for Georgia Public Safety Training Center travels throughout the State of Georgia, holding training classes supporting our community of families. She also role-plays in de-escalation training techniques in the CIT class.

Officer Jaysen Thomas, former Atlanta Police Department and former member of the "HOPE" Team in Atlanta, now coordinates CIT for Georgia Public Safety Training Center. He played intricate roles during his tenure with Atlanta PD. For example, a team of them walked the downtown streets of Atlanta in civilian clothes talking with and assisting the chronic mentally ill, homeless individuals, and military Veteran's years ago. He also role-plays in de-escalation training techniques in the CIT class.

Sgt Renee of the Fayette County Sheriff's Office coordinates CIT and is passionate about supporting and working with the mental health community incarcerated and suicide population. She also role-plays in de-escalation training techniques in the CIT class.

Sgt Faye Spaulding, former Bartow County Police Department, and former Riverdale Georgia Police Department, facilitated and held CIT training classes, bringing in individuals to tell their story of real-life traumatic experiences that impacted them, causing them to have a mental illness diagnosis. She also role-plays in de-escalation training techniques in the CIT class.

Annie Johnson, a sister in faith, shares similar experiences, under- standing we have to continue this journey together because it takes the community of families with prayer and support to hold one another up.

Lonell Speach and I had two children together that are mentioned in these memoirs. Lonell Speach is now deceased and leaves behind other children from another marriage that could also have been born with this disease called mental illness. Unfortunately, there was no diagnosis; with the setback and defeat, he was deprived of the quality of life he could have had. His siblings, like Martha Ann and a host of family members; Cleo, Antrell, and Marci, loved and supported him until his end.

Richard Alston III is a NAMI Dad, and a deceased family member. We married and had one child mentioned in these memoirs. We believe his suffering in silence for many years led him down a path that robbed him of a quality of life that could have lengthened his days had he sought help and support. His sister Sandra, a survivor of the three deceased siblings, was by his side until his end.

Janice Hunt, a sister in faith whom I've known for several years, helped me raise these children and fully understands the ups and downs mental illness brings on the family. We are forever grateful for her.

Dr. Margaret Bristow, Adjunct Professor, storyteller, extraordinaire, and wife, is a family friend I continue to cherish. She has supported us over the years, and for that, I feel blessed by her friendship and love. Minister Beverly Frazier, a sister in faith, has been supportive with prayers and encouraging words during times we have both been in crisis with our families. We have exchanged ideas and resource information for years. Many times, I couldn't have gotten through some tough spots dealing with the mental illness crisis without her listening ear.

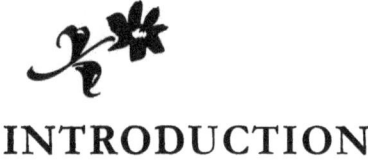

INTRODUCTION

"The Mind is a Terrible Thing To Waste "...a phrase from a commercial years ago advertising College Opportunities to high school graduate students. This is how I would express someone suffering with mental illness. I'm going to expose some real-life situations that have and still are occurring in our family growing up from childhood until now. As you, the reader, walk with me through these pages, I want you to keep an open mind and not look at the morbidity and darkness or helplessness but focus on hopefulness in our situations dealing with mental illness, which I believe some of you can probably relate to as well. Mental illness had such an impact on my life. It's such a severe issue that is genuinely overlooked in our society.

In my opinion, society underrated mental illness, and they still somewhat deny its existence. I never thought once about getting help for Us. I pray through my testimony and my life mission as an advocate, caregiver, and family member with this problem- that in time, people will seek the help they need. God says We are meant to live life and to live it abundantly (John 10:10). This is scripturally given to us. May we seek His guidance and continue to fight the good fight for those who are suffering (1Tim 6:12). LET'S GO!

Mental Illness the Face of Conflict

After many disappointments, frustrations and the feelings of anger that accompany mental illness, I now know that we have to be proactive, vigilant, diligent, and uncover dark spells of gloom from our minds. Because mental illness is the face of conflict, there is such a thing as creative conflict. I know because I sat in several weekly training classes with CIT (Crisis Intervention Team), law enforcement, and mental health medical clinicians. These groups were very informative.

Family Support

I grew up in a dysfunctional family. We all have a little dysfunction in our families. Having an encounter with the Lord made a huge difference in my life, it was very evident because my character began to change and my outlook on life and people changed for the better.

I would later have a conversation with a coworker, not realizing she was prophetic. She asked me to hold out my hands and began to pray with me; she said that the Lord had placed a mantle over me. From that point on, my relationship with the Father in heaven changed. I became ecstatic and began laying hands-on family and friends wanting to heal them. I told my godmother about an experience I had when I touched my family member in a place where they were having pain. The scenario reminded me of the movie "Ghost" when Whoopie allowed the spirit of the ghost to enter her body, and after it left, she felt drained. That's exactly how I felt that day after laying hands on my family member. My godmother, who I affectionately call Ma Gloria said, "baby you, be careful laying hands on everybody."

That statement right there helped me understand to be careful from that point on.

Generational Curses
BLAME OURSELVES (NAMI-Family Perspective)

Inconveniences are sometimes necessary. I heard the Holy Spirit say to me at 4am one morning. The mental illness catalyst and its disease has kept society in denial, tried us, and kept us in the fire with GOD protecting us for many years now. (1 Peter 1:7 NIV) These have come so that the proven genuineness of your faith. The Lord has been really good to our generations with a history of mental illness wreaking havoc on those of us who didn't have the wherewithal to get the help needed 20, 30, 40 years ago. By the grace of God, our family (because some believe mental illness is generational, but not all) through it all; we have survived the trials and tribulations while in the fire. I believe generational curses can be problematic for the children, their children, and so on. It is a continuation of a negative occurrence of the mind that disrupts your blessings but does not kill your promises and purpose from God. (Jeremiah 29:11). I know they can be broken. Why? Because the buck stops here, we are exposing it, fighting it, and embracing it by overcoming stigmas. Taking action by faith, believing that you can overcome this insidious disease is a proactive decision and not a generational curse.

My Successes through these Trails

I'm the 2nd child of seven siblings of the late Sadie Rose, the youngest sibling deceased but not as a result of mental illness. I have a BS in Applied Science in Business Management. Although I worked over 20 years in the educational school system, God was positioning me to do more. What a joy to use my God-given talent, teaching, and work with children. However, I didn't know that my gift to teach and work with children would be very much a part of the mission I'm on with the mental health movement. When I obtained my Bachelor's degree that a college recruiting scout encouraged, only the Lord knew all the intricate details needed to put together this message of encouragement. I had accumulated credits in the field of business in my early years as a young adult, it made sense to finally get this accomplished after 10 years of trying with defeats and setbacks. Later earning a chaplain certification, by the grace of God has been an additional blessing from God. While volunteering for NAMI Georgia's resource helpline, a wife whose spouse was in crisis called, and that's when chaplaincy was born. I share more on my chaplain recruiter experience in another paragraph.

I'm the mother of 4 adult children and 4 grandchildren. After my divorce, I felt so strangely that I was left out to dry. This has been very scary for me and puts me in defense mode often. Nobody but the Lord can help you when things like this begin to happen. What He did for me was send me a large support network of loving friends from professional, non-professionals, ministry community support, and a plethora of friends. I've been involved with NAMI (National Alliance Mental Illness), a grassroots mental health non-profit organization, since 2006. It's been said that God does His best work in the midst of the storms in your life. When I hear this phrase, it gets me moving, so that I don't have time to overthink my life's mission. If I overthink with emotions, I can end up paralyzed with fear of failing and sorrowful for those I love, and never fulfilling the plans and purpose God has for my life, which has been to write this book (Jer 29:11).

About Madea

Our grandmother Mattie Elizabeth lived with us. We called her Madea. As a child, back then, I could see that her behavior was odd in ways that were unexplainable. I remember her being overprotective of us as children. The reason I bring this up is because one day, our dad came to visit, and he had been drinking. You could smell the alcohol. This did not sit well with her. He came into the room I was in, and with excitement, I ran to him but was kept from being held by him. The next thing I knew, our grandmother had slung him into the closet. He stumbled and swiftly ran out the door. I cried because I couldn't go with my daddy. I can't remember much of what happened after that, but in the midst of other incidents, our lives seemed to be in turmoil most of the time.

I loved my grandmother, so in retrospect, in a conversation with one of my siblings, she would have been a powerful woman in her ministry who valued her family. Despite her mental illness, Madea was accomplished in preaching God's Word on Sundays at a church she presided over. I was told by our great aunt, Mable aka Hope, that the Sunday deacons would take the money from her after she had taken up collections to pay the bills to keep the doors of the church open. This act would have broken my heart, which I believe is another obstacle that impacted Madea, causing her to suffer in silence with depression. She was a saleswoman, a mother who loved her daughter (our mother), and a strict grandparent. As children, we experienced some bizarre punishment from her that only by the grace of God we survived. Her behavior caused her to be admitted to Milledgeville Institution.

There's a book that's a must-read entitled "But for the Grace of God" by Dr. Peter G. Crandord, MILLEDGEVILLE! The Inside Story of the World's Largest Insane Asylum, and although the dates are around 1842-1952, our grandmother must have been in that population back then during the 1930-40s era. Not sure how long, but we knew she had been to Milledgeville Mental Institution by the way she responded when she was released into our mother's care. Our grandmother didn't respond to us the same after returning home because of the "shock treatments" they said she received.

Madea had some good days, I remember her teaching us a song. It sounded like the sinner's prayer that went, "O Lord Jesus be merciful unto me, come into my heart and save me today, I take Jesus as my personal Lord Savior Amen, and Amen. She also would chant "Jesus" in a song over and over, sitting on the edge of her bed with tears rolling down her cheeks. I recall peeking around the corner of her bedroom sometimes just to watch her. She never moved from that spot some days, but I recall her routine was caring for us, cooking, and having Bible lessons.

When I feel down in my spirit or confused about a decision to make in my life concerning anything, this sets off the anxiety in me. Madea's "Jesus" chant rings out in my head, and over and over again, I say it. You could say it's like a soothing balm.

During my high school years as a senior, we had memory books (like today's yearbooks). I had my friends and teachers sign. One particular teacher grabbed my attention because she was completely honest with me about my behavior and attitude. She told me that I would succeed in life but that I had to stop being so hateful. I was oblivious to what she meant because I couldn't see the irritable, confused and frustrated young teenager she saw. I didn't realize that what we endured (my siblings and I) would affect us years into our adult life. I can only speak of my experience from this point, although, I do understand that all have been affected in some way.

Madea's Daughter-our mother

Our Mother, Sadie Rose was an only child. She was a "cutter" (suicidal) and was institutionalized in her early twenties leaving us to be cared for by relatives (aunts, uncles, and cousins). It was very hard being away from our mother, and I'm certain it impacted us negatively in some aspects. Although it kept us out of foster care, it was very hard on us as young children. We all know there's nothing like having the security of being with your mother and father. We returned home in mother's care after she had gotten better. I recall accurate stories told by her of her being a depressed soul. I heard about her childhood struggles, and troubles inflicted after being sent on an errand to pick up a package, she was assaulted by an adult male. She returned home with blood all over her dress. She was whipped by her mother (our grandmother), leaving her filled with feelings of shame, confusion, anger, and frustration. After our mother married our father, who was a military veteran, he would come home and they would drink alcohol, fight and make babies. This impacted us all nega- tively, so our father was banned by our grandmother from ever coming around us again when I was 5 years old.

Now over 40 years later, mental illness shows up at my doorstep, something I didn't raise my hand for, and since being catapulted into it, I learned to accept it. While being willing to hear from God in this matter was hard at times because I was so angry, which kept me out of the will of God, often taking matters into my own hands, I couldn't hear the lessons I needed to learn in all this. Humbly I needed to walk with obedience to God, which was not one of my strong points.

I realized when your mind is messed up, nobody but the person going through it suffers most, and realize I the family was suffering too. It took our peace away, and the spirit of confusion wreaked havoc on us.

One sermon I remember the pastor, TJ McBride at our church, Tabernacle of Praise Church International, spoke on Faith Focus Principles, the sermon gave me a double dose of confirmation. I realized not only do I need education from a practical standpoint, but I also need the Holy Spirit to continue teaching me how to build up my most holy faith (1Tim 4:7). This journey is never-ending, and it is a marathon, not a sprint (Dr. Lloyd Sederer YouTube Ted X).

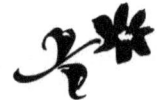

STATEMENT OF SUPPORT

I've known Chaplain Delora for over 10 years. I've seen her fight tirelessly for her adult children's recovery, intervene with families in crisis, share her story in the community public's eye, and advocate for countless individuals with mental illness. She has a wealth of experience, and a plethora of knowledge that I know will help you and your loved ones. In the past, we had conversations about her book. One day during a phone conversation, she asked for an acronym of her children's first initials JNPA...I blurted out, "Just No Problem Advocating". I've seen this family make milestones in their lives, and sharing their stories takes great courage. I tell people, "When You Know Better You Do Better".

Reading this book will give you insight that I hope will enable you to do better. Ms. Selina Beene

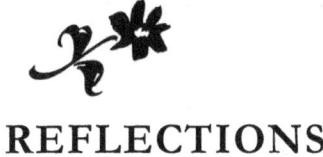

REFLECTIONS

From Our Son

My life started off very distorted. My thinking had been delusional ever since I was a child. After going to prison for becoming a criminal with a self-centered mindset. I was hearing voices. I didn't hear them all the time, but every now and then and when I heard them, they told me things like I could do what I wanted to do, and that it didn't matter how other people looked at me, and that I was better than other people. I'm thankful when I went to prison, the experiences I went through gave me the dose of reality that I needed because I was so out of touch with who I was. I thought I could create things with just mere words that came out of my mouth (which is true because there is power in words). The words I used impacted my life negatively, landing me in all sorts of trouble. I was given medication because of my violent nature and rebellious attitude that accompanied my belief system around my mental issues while locked up. I always felt that I was at war with my life, only to find out later that self-medication was the cure-all sending me in a downward spiral to the disease of addiction.

So as time went along and I began to get older, the voices that I heard began to haunt me, and these voices took over my actions when I used drugs or became trapped in my anger. I had no control and became so impulsive in my behavior that violence toward myself and others was all I knew, so I used drugs to keep myself calm. I could not understand my hate for the police; I felt they were out to get me because I was oblivious to the fact that breaking the law would have them get me. I saw correction officers murder a friend in prison; so I carried that anger with me, and I acted out on it even as years went by. This incident plays repeatedly in my head today as if it had just taken place yesterday. I was diagnosed with PTSD after witnessing this trauma, later my clinical diagnosis Paranoid Schizophrenia, Borderline Personality Disorder, Psychotic (NOS), and depression as my label. I took a vast assortment of medications. Sometimes I amped up the situation while incarcerated just to get more medications because my mind was damaged and I held onto so much negative stuff. I never thought that I could make it out. Now here I sit through the voice of my mom telling you, the reader, that there is HOPE and whatever you do, never give up on you. I stopped hearing voices, and God has been the light of my life daily.

From Our 1st Daughter

Being a mental health individual has been a struggle most of my life since I was a child. I experienced obstacles and hardships through my ability to learn and get along with others. I can't remember how old I was when the noise in my head began. The images of seeing things, the mood swings, and the depressive modes that I live in puts my life, my world, and my behavior in a state of turmoil all the time. Each day of my life consist of me trying to balance my activities and medication, it's an ongoing conflict that causes me to be manic in spending and overeating.

The side effects from the psychotropic medication I have to take have not cured me. It suppresses my mental state so I can sleep without interruption. I have been without medication off and on because I can't afford it sometimes. I have developed other health issues because I don't always eat right, putting my physical -well-being at risk. The flip side of it all is that with self-willingness to pray, the support and prayers of my mother and father; has encouraged me to live my life with the determination to recover by setting goals and making healthy choices for myself. With God's help, I will win, no matter how long it takes.

From Our 2nd Daughter

This is an apology letter she wrote on January 28, 2021, after a bad episode of conflict between us.

> Dear Momma, it's your 2nd daughter; first, I want to say I do apologize for swearing at my earth mother, an older Black woman. This is wrong...I know I have not been the best daughter, but it is not about me. I can clearly see you need assistance with your recov- ery from your eye surgery procedure. I am appalled at your lack of support right now. I could not sleep last night, and I felt so convicted by God yesterday that no one has brought you any flowers or expressed outward love towards you. As our mother, I am here for you for

anything that you may need, especially in your time of need of healing, and recovery. I will not abandon you like this; it is wrong in God's eyes. I will also, no matter how long it takes, be staying here with my girls. I am not having them live in a hotel or shelter. I am staying at your house until I secure my own house for you two precious grand girls whom they call Grand D. I am here for you if you need me.

I will never cuss at my mother again and I will work with the Lord on how to honor and respect my Mom. Until I truly learn how to honor her and be a blessing to her. I will stay in your home until I get it right. Again, I cannot be moved by others' behavior in this house. I am not Bi-polar, but I have bouts of Bi-polar. So, this is why I am not going anywhere with my two little girls with no plan and no money. So, in closing, if you need anything, please let me know. Lovingly In Christ Jesus, Your 2nd daughter.

From Our 3rd Daughter

As the youngest of our mom's 4 children, I have seen her hold up under some real hard situations dealing with mental illness. My eyes have seen a lot of crazy situations that made me flee when I saw my older sibling's problems with mental illness. I tried to get as far South going to college there to never return to the city I grew up in and loved. I married and had 2 children miscarrying one. Starting my own family later to learn that the struggles in my life would take me to a place where I was about to give up hope and throw my life away. After my mother and I had a conversation- that day sitting in my car, she listened while I cried then reminded me of who I was and that I was that very strong, gifted, and talented young woman that had a life worth living and fighting for. All praises and glory to God for our/my mother for her strength, prayers, and determination to see this book come to reality. She is my SHERO, and I pray that her memoirs will help others the way she has helped me.

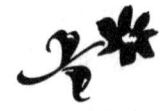

CHAPTER 1

Clueless

I have not one, two, three, but four children, three of them who have been clinically diagnosed and the fourth one who refused to hear a diagnosis. I won't use their names but instead will refer to her as daughter #1 etc. I decline to give their diagnosis because I don't want readers to focus so much on the diagnosis. After all, they are not their diagnoses, but people with a human condition that limits their sound reasoning and decision making. Daughter #1 first "Dark days' ' began when she was 7 or 8 years old, Back then or maybe sooner. One day, I remember being called into the school she attended by the school administrator. As I entered the room, she sternly spoke, "You sit down right now"? I was nervous, startled and clueless at what she was about to tell me. She said that my daughter was having loud outbursts, tantrums, turning over desks and that whatever her father and I were doing needed to stop because it was ruining her. I couldn't handle this report, so I walked away feeling so ashamed, guilty, afraid, and con- fused about what to do. My inadequacy to comprehend this process led me to do nothing about it, and her behavior continued. Her dad James Alfred has been a significant part of her life and a wonderful supporter since day one. It wasn't always positive outcomes because we didn't understand how to handle what would come. He had been dealing with the same issues on his side of the family and understood the behavior challenges better than I did at that time. Over the years, society has changed the names for folks like us, and that name is caregivers and enablers. Her father and I had done a great job at being both caregivers and enablers back then because we loved her. When our daughter was school age, she would sing out her bedroom window to our neighbor's kids the R&B duet-how do you keep the music playing, (with the words-with any luck then I suppose, the music never ends). I think back then, that was how she would soothe herself by singing to cope, whether it was R&B or gospel. She sang the Lord's Prayer at our United Methodist Women's Conference as a teenager. I was proud of her magnificent voice because she could sing so pretty.

Later on, through middle school years, she struggled with her mental illness, which we didn't know what to call it then. More of the same continued throughout high school; the signs and symptoms were isolating myself, sleeping, compulsive eating, and irritability. Barely making it by the "skin of her teeth" she graduated from high school. She learned the language Arabic very well, which I found out later, and with all that was going on with her, which was phenomenal. She had an Asian friend she was fond of. She told her siblings during that time about her problem, but they kept it a secret for several years, and I didn't become fully aware until much later. On her 18th birthday, her father and I gave her a party at the Embassy Suites Hotel, where we invited most of her cousins, the twins, some other family members, classmates, and friends. She seemed so happy, and I thought this "quick fix" would help her pull herself together, so to speak.

But after it was over, she reverted back into her shell and familiar patterns of irritability, sleeping, and isolation. Looking back, there were the warning signs back then in the 80's and 90's era, but I treated her like a normal child. People with diagnoses can appear to be lazy or just don't feel like doing anything; these are called symptoms I would learn later on. Because of the lack of understanding and educational knowledge about mental illness, terms like (psychosis), a term I was oblivious to, would help us understand what we were dealing with, and it would follow her into college. We submitted her application on the recommendation of our pastor because the church supported higher education. She got accepted for the scholarship at a 2-year college, an hour's drive from home in a small town in Georgia. Her silver lining had appeared and in her 2nd year college, she joined the singing ensemble where each member of the group received a plaque with their own name on it for outstanding performance.

  I remember how proud she was, but not long after this, the symp- toms started again, and she became progressively worse. Some of the signs were phone calls home of her telling us she was hearing voices, and that her roommate was plotting to put things in her luggage bags. She went on to describe seeing blood and strange symbols outside her window. I began to freak out and became frustrated, explaining to her that if this continued, she would have to come home. What made matters worse, I knew she needed to seek counseling there first, but with no diagnoses or medication, she couldn't explain to them what to expect, which made matters worse. I knew nothing of how to go about getting her help with medication. She struggled academically and was told that because it was a two-year college, she could run into student loan debt past the two-year required curriculum. She ended up going back and forth with episodes entering into her 3rd year. By this time, her scholarship money had run out. I stepped in at this point because she was getting worse and told her we had to withdraw her and find other alternatives for her education. At this point, you can guess what happened next; that's right, I was the blame for ruining her college career, and she was angry at me, causing us to have heated arguments.

DON'T GET INTO FIGHTS (Dr. Lloyd Sederer You-Tube-Ted Talks) Not getting into verbal fights was getting harder. She would even- tually ostracize herself after a "shouting match" with me. The chemical imbalance led her down a slippery slope and miserable path of isolation and more of the same symptoms of hearing voices and seeing strange images.

By the time she was 21 years old, I think she ended up leaving home to live with other family members. Then the phone calls started coming asking me questions trying to understand her behavior. With no diagnosis or medication yet, we would all suffer miserably with her for several years. We never became physical because I wouldn't allow myself to lose self-control that way, but I would be very frustrated, sad, and angry. She was taken to the psychiatrist by her cousins once, and the doctor summed it up with comments like "when her backs against the wall," she falls apart.

Unfortunately, people with mental diagnoses are viewed negatively. Comments like, they're probably just mad or depressed because things aren't going their way or they just need a swift kick in the pants are all too familiar derogatories.

I worried a lot about her and prayed she would make it. About this time, there was an influx of homelessness that took downtown Atlanta by surprise. It was happening around the time that Atlanta had historically been selected to hold the 1996 Olympics Games. I'm now hearing over 23 years later how the political and administrative folks covered up the problem by buying the mentally challenged homeless people "tuxedos" to keep down embarrassment and sending this population somewhere other than downtown.

The fact that my child was a female, we were very concerned about her state and well-being, and there were times I would drive to work seeing homeless people on the streets. Sometimes asking her father if he had seen her, he would mention that he would run into her not far from where he was living and would give her a lift home and anything else she needed.

Then one sunny day, our daughter knocked on our door, standing with grocery bags dressed in a red sweat shirt and beige khaki pants and with braided hair; I'll never forget it. She looked well, but I knew she was struggling. I invited her in and embraced her with a big hug, asking her where she had been all this time? She had tears in her eyes explaining what she could. From that day, as we reunited, I got busy going to her place where she lived with a young couple with 2 children that were renting her a basement apartment.

As I sat and listened, the young woman told me what they had observed. She had held down a job at the Hartsfield Jackson International Airport all that time to support herself. The landlord, a very sweet and concerned soul, stated that our daughter needed to get medical and professional help, not in those words but that she also needed my help. All the while, our daughter lived there as a tenant with this married couple and their 2 children; they never said they were afraid of her. I got busy and learned about the mental health system by making a phone call to the Access line I remember calling back then, which is called BHL (Behavioral Health Link) Georgia Crisis & Access Line today. The lady on the other end listened to me and then asked what was my daughter's main concern, and I told her 3 things. 1) how she was to pay her bills, 2) a place to stay, 3) and food to eat. She then said I had to take her to the ER (Emergency Receiving Facility) hospital and get her admitted to be assessed and tell her that she could get a check if she let them help her. The statement made by intake staff shocked me; little did I know that the process would turn out to be grueling. I was desperate to get help for her, so I did what she said. The requirements for disability for mental illness were 2 years of homelessness and being on medication to create a paper trail. I became relieved but frustrated at the same time for what I was about to endure. Now, keep in mind that I'm a mother desperately seeking to help her daughter, and following mental health system protocol. After telling us of this lengthy waiting process, I was to take her to a day shelter where you had to get out to go to work during the day and sleep in at night. Now keep in mind she has an illness with no diagnosis and no medication yet, so her days were spent walking up and down the street all day.

One bitterly cold winter day, I got a call from a resident at the shelter telling me he left 8 hours ago to work and saw her still walking up and down the road in a daze after returning to the shelter. He then said he felt very bad for her and asked me to please come and get her. I broke down and cried, asked my job if I could attend to a family emergency, and went to pick her up. I resented the mental health system and felt this was a horrible way to enter into it.

The next step was when I made a decision to pack her suitcase, taking her to the local CSB (Community Service Board) in the county where I explained to my daughter that we had to get her accepted and assessed and to not let them turn her away. It was our only hope. Not long after dropping her off, before I could get in the door of my home, the phone rang. There was a woman on the other end yelling at me telling me I abandoned my daughter, I replied, "ma'am how do you abandon a 26-year-old adult at a facility that helps people with mental illness? Well, you know what would have happened if she had come back home with me, we wouldn't have gotten the help she needed. The staff and I continued to go back and forth until I shouted, this is what we lobby for, and before I knew it, the staff worker took her in, and her process began. My daughter got her medication, therapy, housing to a group home, living with 4 roommates. Then this dwindled down to finally ending up on her own. She has always been medication compliant, but as you read earlier, she can't always afford her medication, putting her in crisis periodically. Today she drives a car and works a very good full-time job taking care of people that are disabled. Has it been easy? The answer is NO. We still get in crisis sometimes but thank God we never gave up.

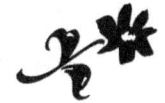

CHAPTER 2

Caught off Guard

DENY WARNING SIGNS (NAMI-Family Perspective)

I was caught off guard; Daughter #2 a "Cum Laude", quiet, passive-aggressive, was stricken with this illness. I would later learn that she had told her oldest sister in secret, "Don't tell mom, but I think I'm like you". We have to pay attention to our children during our busy lives because they have secrets right under your nose in your home. Daughter #2 got along well with her siblings, so they never gave me a reason to question their relationships with each other. They hid her mental illness from me, and as I would learn much later, she became progressively worse because she had not been diagnosed or on medication yet. Seeing this made me want to scream, but there isn't much I could do. I could see that I had been in denial all along. I thought this just can't be true. I assumed her picking at her food and being underweight was just part of her being studious and stressed out about college. She was always what you would consider a high achiever.

I remember her kindergarten teacher telling me at a school event she was bright and would go very far in school. This brought tears to my eyes, and I was ecstatic with excitement to watch her academic years soar to the level she achieved. I can count the number of times she was spanked as a child. She was always quiet, never saying much, her siblings would talk over her in conversations, and she would just sit there. Growing up she made straight A's, and if she made a "B", she would strive harder to get that A grade. In Middle School, she did exceptionally well and went on to do even better upon entering high school. She graduated receiving $10,000 in scholarship from school and $3600 more from our local United Methodist Church. She got 4 offers to colleges and decided to pursue the one that offered chiropractic licensing and worked very hard to succeed academically until the awful news came that the university had gotten into a financial predicament, forcing students to find alternative options to finish their college studies. She wouldn't allow that to become an obstacle, so she immediately went on to enroll in Georgia State University, got accepted, and the rest was history. Upon graduating from college, she earned "Cum Laude " and finished debt-free from student loans. Around age 25, we started talking to her about her goals and what she wanted to do with her degree. Moving into her own apartment was a dream. We agreed that she would contact her college friend, who was an artist. They became roommates making plans to share an apartment. Our daughter's friend had her parents come over and pray for them in the apartment. Right after her move, she had a psychotic break, I believe, and her nightmare began. One morning at 1:00am, she told the roommate that someone was trying to break into the apartment and that they needed to get out right away. I got a call, not sure which came first whether it was her roommate's parents or our daughter telling us what happened.

We were all devastated, and this threw us into a state of panic and disbelief. Prior to this incident, I should have noticed the signs and symptoms she was having. She would drive somewhere and not be able to drive back to her destination or figure out where and ask me to come and get her. But I missed all of the warning signs. After bringing her back home, our nightmare of "Dark days' ' had already begun. I remember telling her that everyone could see there was a problem with her but herself, and she covered her mouth in shock.

At this point, mental illness began to cause my family to question what was going on as if I had caused this terrible disease, which strained my marriage as well. Our oldest sibling said in a phone conversation when I told her what was happening, and she shouted, "I'm not dealing with generational people. I thought to myself, what is she talking about? Then I started to take a look at our family history. Our grandmother suffered, and our mother had a mental illness.

One day feeling that my family had a generational curse I went off the deep end buying books on spiritual warfare strategies. It gave information on how to protect yourself, your family, and if you read it for 30 days, you will begin to see the results. Boy, did I see results. I could see the demons beginning to manifest before my eyes one night around midnight while praying alone in my small office in our home. Sounds ``spooky", well it was. The author of the book said that's when the dark worshipers, divination, and incantations are doing their "bubble bubble toil and trouble".

After this, I realized that you don't go into warfare alone; second it helps to have another believer in agreement with you.

God stepped in through a couple of intercessors one day through a co-worker who I would meet with in an empty classroom. She called her cousin in another state. We began to pray over the phone then something very interesting started to happen. The cousin began to prophesy. I listened to her say, "every time I move on it you put your mouth on it, take your mouth off of it". I didn't even realize God was listening. This was startling and very unexpected. I walked away weeping with all kinds of mixed emotions.

My next step was to take her to the CSB in our local county, to start the same situation that I mentioned earlier with daughter #1; homelessness, which meant another shelter, proof of being on medication for 2 years and in and out of mental facilities (Yikes). During our visit with the intake nurse, daughter#2 sat across from her while the nurse explained that she was not "crazy" but had a chemical imbalance. At that moment, she stood up and replied, "I was born into this," and we both began to weep.

We took the following steps and fearfully headed to a shelter which went very bad, I would learn later. The staff said that there was no place for her or to find a women's shelter for her. I've lost track of the series of events that took place because of the stress during this time and the order in which they came. Later after an episode at home, another round at a mental institution, would again lead me to get her help. I received a call from the onsite social worker telling me that I needed to come in to talk to daughter #2 because she was hostile, and was using profane language. I had to get her to calm down otherwise, they couldn't help her. She then told me that I needed to keep myself together because our daughter needed my help handing me a NAMI pamphlet.

There was a physical assault committed by the staff at that facility. I learned about it later from our daughter #2. It was about how two workers took punches, hitting her in the chest multiple times. It angered and hurt me that she had endured this type of treatment and concluded that was probably why she wouldn't cooperate with the treatment team. This criminal act should have been reported, but I didn't find out from her until sometime later. It was while having a talk trying to help her understand that she was loved and important to God, and that I did what the mental health system told me to do. This abuse would make her more angry and bitter. I tried to convince her that we were helping her, not hurting her. I told her I was sorry about what happened and I wish she had told me sooner. She replied, "everyone else abuses me", why should I care, or something along those lines.

I became disgusted and angry with the mental health system, which left me feeling so powerless. I was desperate, so I followed up on the advice of the social worker at that mental institution. I contacted NAMI, and they recommended I go to my local family support group in my county. There I met other family members like me that were coping by attending the family support groups. Later on, the NAMI movement started putting changes in place, giving us a positive model listing several principles and guidelines to use. They said they wanted families to begin focusing on solutions rather than their family member's problems at the meetings. Two NAMI family members came up to train me. They were sisters (Mimi & Sue) from Columbus, Georgia. They explained to me that they knew how I felt having dealt with mental illness themselves in their family. They said to me, "We know you feel like the wheels have fallen off", and it did.

My drive to continue was restored with their commitment, support, and encouraging words. I took the information and ran with it. I continued to attend family support meetings regularly and attended training offered at our state-level NAMI office. Attending the NAMI National Convention was an experience that showed me how the medical professionals and families come together for a cause that's powerful.

I met "The Soloist" (Nathaniel Ayers) and the news reporter while riding in an elevator at the Conference. Mr. Ayers' story was turned into a movie-Journey from Juilliard to Skid Row starring popular actors, Jamie Fox and Robert Downy Jr. The high points in this journey still could not outweigh the struggles, but I was so grateful and honored to be at the convention. I had a talk with my daughter one day. She was crying and seemed depressed, then asked, "Mom, do you think I'll ever get married or have children? " As we sat down on her bedroom floor, I told her Yes, but the truth was that I really didn't know. A few years later, God smiled on her, and she met the man she would marry at the treatment facility she attended. They had the most beautiful wedding. She looked stunning, had her two sisters in the wedding, and her step dad gave her away. However, to my surprise, I was not invited. I was caught off guard; I wanted to see our daughter walk down that aisle. Realizing she was not thinking clearly, I attended the wedding along with her brother, who also was not invited. It turned into a Tyler Perry moment when the preacher asked if anyone objected to this marriage; her brother jumped up and grabbed the microphone expressing, while weeping of course, that he wanted to give her away.

This is another example of what mental illness can do to a family when the soul suffering is angry or not thinking clearly about others' feelings. Bernadine, Aaron, and Steve, our in-laws who have been part of our support system, and a very important intricate part of the family in this process, have embraced our daughter. Bernadine once said to me if I recall correctly, they loved her as their own. But over the course of time, that has changed. We have tension between us, and it's very sad to say that the enemy thinks he has won when we don't come together in love. My daughter and her husband have two beautiful little girls. It truly does take the village to help raise our granddaughters, whos at the time of writing this book was, 8yrs and 4yrs, and to celebrate their lives; praying that the inevitable won't happen to them. You may be asking, are the children aware of what's going on? The answer is yes, and I don't hide it from them. I had a conversation with an Attorney and a NAMI dad one day. They helped me to understand many of my frustrations with mental illness and its constant interruptions. Their words to me, "you're a caregiver, and it's very difficult at times raising children with parents that are sick, but the kids get hip to what's going on after a while".

 We are in the DFACS system now with support to get them and myself counseling. The next hardest thing I've had to do is take custody of my granddaughters, so they wouldn't end up in the system as foster kids. We're not the only family addressing issues like these situations that make the children blurt out in public, saying things like, my mommy doesn't want me, or I want mommy to stop having crying spells. It's tough, and the best thing to do is hold the children and tell them it's okay to want mommy, so let's pray for her.

 Our second daughter is in crisis again as I type these words. She moved out again and made several attempts trying to manage her illness without medication. She left her children and now her husband. I'm grateful God gives me the strength to support and raise my grandkids, so they don't end up in the system. I received a call from a public defender who said our daughter was being detained for locking a restroom door and refusing to come out, or let others enter at a local establishment. We concluded she was trying to keep herself safe while being on the streets during the early hours of the morning. Engaging her in conversation while being held, the public defender said she noticed she seemed disoriented. Our daughter told her she was scared. Not sure how long she could be detained; the best recourse was looking for a place to transition her because to bring her back into the home would be more of the same conflict.

(2 Corinth 4:8-12) We are hard-pressed on every side, but not crushed, perplexed, but not in despair, persecuted, but not abandoned, struck down but not destroyed. I would hold onto this scripture years later as my ministry developed that the Lord gave me- encouraging me to run on.

CHAPTER 3

A Vicious Cycle of Mental Illness

LEARN THE MENTAL HEALTH SYSTEM
(Dr. Lloyd Sederer YouTube-Ted Talks)

My only adult son is very smart as well, and could pass a class without attending every day. However, he could not sit still in the classroom to finish assignments. The behaviors of Mental Illness would be the biggest downfall in his academic learning career. He has his own conspiracy theory. He ended up in the penile system; as a result of his missed diagnosis, he was left struggling for years without us being aware. I thought his overactive behavior at age 5 was normal. Someone hinted that he could have ADHD, but I didn't follow through the process to get him tested because I didn't know where to start. I was paranoid about putting him on medication at a young age. I got calls from the teacher at his school relaying instances about his pre- cocious acts (talkativeness), being a distraction to the other students, and not staying in his seat. Being the only boy of three girls, I'm sure he felt outnumbered, so I concluded that was why he felt he had to act out to get the extra attention. I would have him with me a lot of times when running errands to make him feel that he could be a team leader. I contacted various agencies that assisted the youth such as Big Bros/Sisters, CHAMPS, a youth mentoring organization that assists with preparing young boys to be successful students, and they had a job-focused curriculum for at-risk youth. When he was about nine years old, we would be at a family function, and he would disappear for a while and eventually show up later. When asked where he had been, he would tell stories about being captured by aliens and say strange names of the thing that took him off somewhere. I always thought he was trying to humor us because he liked to make his sisters laugh with his made-up stories to get attention.

Still denying warning signs, we would later learn that our son was suffering from delusions. I had family friends who mentored our son, we affectionately called them Papa George and Darryl. This made him happy for a while, but because of his dad's absence, the void remained. I recall when he was still school age, he would get on the landline home phone during the early morning hours after everyone in the house was asleep, talking on the phone soliciting inappropriate conversations with an adult. He was only 11years old then. I caught it just in time, and his behind was mine. He got a lot of spankings for his bad behaviors, but never putting 2 and 2 together would later come back to haunt me. I wanted the best for him and was determined he would not get mixed up with the wrong crowd or end up in the juvenile system.

However, the inevitable did happen. I asked his sisters when they noticed he was starting to change, and one of them said, "when we moved to this neighborhood, mama". We lived in a complex where the economic disparity was not good for a single parent raising a young male child. Around the early to mid-'90s if the young males didn't have consistency with positive male role models, it was easy to get caught up in peer pressure and negative influence. Over a period of time, he became hostile and irritable, causing him to mess around with alcohol and street drugs. I saw his life spinning out of control and did not know what to do. I felt helpless, frustrated, angry, and very scared for him. I remember an instance where he had cursed the neighbor in the same complex that lived across from us. She had it in for him, and so did I. So, one day, because he was always on the run, I told her to let me know when she saw him. She did, we jumped and held him. The neighbor sneaked and bit my son. I learned this after he got into the police car crying. I was scolding him when he admitted he was not crying because he was going to juvenile, but it was because the neighbor had bitten a plug out of him. That didn't sit well with me, and I had resentment towards her.

    I confronted her, and her reply was, I bite my children when they are being bad". We didn't press charges, but in the back of my mind, I concluded she had issues if she was biting children. The police drove him away that day, and from then on, he was in and out of the juvenile system. Like most parents, I wanted the best for him and was determined he would not end up in the penile system; however, the inevitable would happen. The mistakes he made later as a teen would later run him into more trouble with the law. He eventually landed himself in prison doing time served (10yrs) which was part of a plea bargain of a 20-year sentence that was reduced only by the Grace of God. Ten years of his life were carved away from him, missing family birthdays, holidays, etc.

    Five, maybe six years into his sentence, I had a friend, Minister Cox, who introduced me to a family prison ministry called Kairos Outside. The website address is www.mykairos.org.

There are Kairos ministries inside too. They have an awesome weekend of celebrating families with loved ones that are incarcerated. I was so moved emotionally by the love displayed by these women I met for the first time, volunteering their time to ensure we felt loved and appreci- ated for everything we go through when our loved ones are absent for long periods. The Lord knew what I needed to help get through some tough spots when the special occasions would come around; all praise and Glory to God for connecting me to this ministry of women that showed an abundance of love in a weekend retreat. What a special gift that entailed celebrating every special occasion that our son missed.

Meanwhile, I got a call one day from the psychiatric nurse because he was in some trouble, something to do with him running into a gang fight instead of running away from it and climbing the walls to the ceiling, which led the correction officer to take notice. They could only imagine what it must have been like for them to talk him down to do an intervention. Staff led him to see a psychiatrist at the prison, where they dug deep into his past history. This opened up his can of worms, as he began telling them what was wrong with him.

I got a call one day, and the conversation from the doctor on the other end went something like this "Mom, did you know your son was suffering from a mental illness"? In that moment of disbelief, I started to weep and feel very helpless because I was limited to what I could do for him while incarcerated. She went on to say they did an assessment history of our son's life experiences growing up. Then they asked me, did you know that your son has been hearing voices since he was 4 years old? Silent with disbelief, I don't remember my response except feeling fear in its darkest form along with sadness. This vicious cycle of mental illness had overtaken him and us by surprise, leaving me with no recourse of action. He was incarcerated and in the hands of the system. She said when he admitted he had a mental illness diagnosis, tears rolled down his face while explaining the voices in his head that he had been hearing since the age of 4. This would explain the anger and frustration he had been dealing with most of his childhood until now. It all started to make sense with the behavior he displayed. His struggles growing up as a youth, and to make matters worse, we didn't know that he was suffering with a mental illness because he never disclosed it to anyone until he was incarcerated.

After that, they put him on medication, and the crisis phone calls would come frequently. All I knew to do was what he requested, and that would be to ask the warden to have him transferred because he was paranoid about someone out to get him; this went on repeatedly. This kept me in a state of panic and worry all the time. When he was released in 2009, the next five years of his life would be a nightmare. I remember telling him I couldn't bring him home because I was afraid of the conflict between him and his stepdad. Instead, I put him up at an extended stay hotel because I knew it would be hard adjusting as he displayed a lot of pinned-up anger. After saying those words to him that evening and then dropping him off, I saw a very frustrated young man walk away with his hands in his pocket disappearing in the dark of the night.

I felt very bad and guilty because I had to leave him there. From then on, he would have to find his own way of making a life for himself. I continued to learn the mental health system through advocacy, attending meetings, and helping other families God would send my way. Even in the midst of all the chaos going on in our lives, I had to keep going. I already knew the steps to take homelessness, then getting him to stay on his medication and psychotherapy. He had his own conspiracy theory about taking medication, telling me that taking the medication would make him feel very sleepy, gain weight and cause side effects like type 2 diabetes. We failed miserably over the years; he had weight gain and said he didn't like the way the medication made him feel or the side effects that affected his manhood.

Later on, he would take matters into his own hands by self-medicating using drugs to cope. This would put him in crisis often. I recall one really bad situation that I considered the worst, where he was using drugs and running with people that meant to harm him. We all know street drugs are a death sentence within themselves. An altercation broke out between him and another fellow one night. It turned into a brutal fight where his attacker broke a glass bottle and cut up his face. He didn't come to me right away but went to a friend and called me, weeping, saying, "It was my fault, Mama, it was my fault". He stayed with them for a while until he healed, but that didn't stop him. He kept getting into more fights using drugs, and being attacked to the point where the person involved would try to kill him. In one instance, the attacker took an ice pick, stabbing the side of his head near his skull. He is blessed to be alive. These incidents kept my nerves on edge and kept me stressed out. Through all of this, we would find recovery programs, but he would not stay and would run away back to the drug traps.

It got so bad I began to question God, asking, "Is he going to make it"? It would take more trials of getting him out of tight situations to not seeing or hearing from him until one day, finally, things began to look up. Our son confessed later on that the voices in his head stopped as he got older. The struggles with staying clean and sober were no longer an option. He was getting tired of not having and living the way he was with no structure or goals set for himself to recover. It was a miracle happening right before our eyes.

Today even with his track record, this young man has recovered. He works for a company that allows him to travel to different states even in the midst of this Pandemic (COVID-19). He takes care of himself through a network of support from mutual friends that care about his well-being.

All the heartbreaks and maltreatment from bad people ceased. He has also overcome his fear of policemen because of the negative run-ins with them times past. He tells his story of how that officer confronted him one day while he was on the streets, walking around looking down. The policeman he remembers very well as he recalled and asked him, "Man, are you alright?" At that moment, he said that he must have been a CIT (Crisis Intervention Team Officer) because of his approach and what he said. He took him to the ER (Emergency Receiving Unit) and got him on his medication again. The program IOOV (In Our Own Voice under NAMI) at the CIT Training has afforded our young man on several occasions to tell his story, and he ends with giving a handshake to the officers and thanking them for their service.

Because "Recovery is Good Business", God helped him put his life on track with gainful employment with a major company making a lucrative salary. Our son is also responsible for funding this book project, sending a team of professional business people to manage the marketing phase of this project which has been a huge blessing. I give praise and the glory to Father in Heaven for it all. Our son continues to take care of his mind attending meetings and talking with his support network of those that believe in him. He has a bright future because we believe in God and what He has promised this young man. Our son's desire is to marry and have children someday, and that's our prayer for him too, as he continues to submit himself to God, the light of his life. (Jeremiah 29:1) For I know the thoughts that I think toward you, saith the Lord, thoughts of peace, and not of evil to give you an expected end.

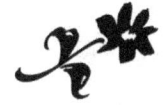

CHAPTER 4

Blindsided

WONDER WHAT CAUSED THE ILLNESS
(NAMI Family Perspective Talk)

Lastly, the adult daughter #3, the 4th child, caught me totally by surprise when she opened up about her situation and feelings that she would articulate while spending time with her this past Mother's Day 2021 during this Pandemic. I could see exchanging tokens of love meant a lot when I visited her. Because she's my youngest, I've tried to protect and ensure her future would not take the course her siblings did, that she would be fine getting through her life without mental illness interruption. She showed no signs or symptoms like her siblings except sadness (depression) which we all experience from time to time in our lives. Trying to handle so much turmoil overwhelmed her, I'm sure. In kindergarten, she had the ability to take charge, and her first experience with her kindergarten teacher would be remarkably remembered. She praised her for being her best student and leader in the class. She then began to tear up when I announced that she was being transferred to the school with her older siblings. Feeling very guilty for taking her away was a tough decision that had to be made. I had no idea she had this type of influence at 5 years of age. If I could change things, I would have left her there and made the sacrifice to transport her back there with her former kindergarten teacher and her siblings to the new school. Her experience at the new elementary school would go over well after she settled in, which took some time but eventually, we all assembled. Years later, she's sharing a memory that she saw at age five behavior from one of her siblings, accusing the other sibling of putting hair on her pillow. The other sibling would then retaliate, doing the same thing but excessively putting hair on her pillow. God only knows how much she's seen, causing her to question whether it was ok to behave this way.

Wondering what caused the illness caused her to shut down emotionally and not talking it out later has impacted her future with feelings of uncertainty, sadness, and disappointment. She recently opened up about her adolescent years. She thanked me for finding a middle school and enrolling there, giving her a chance to grow. She would later take a class trip to Washington D.C. that she still talks about today and the educational learning of how it affected her attitude about culture. She had a very good relationship with her dad, but unless it was initiated, he was not consistently involved in her academia. She graduated from high school, but her dad was a no-show after promising he would. The look I saw on her face that day and seeing how she buckled in her knees, falling to the floor weeping, left me feeling awful. Another frightening experience she had, along with disappoint- ment, was when I forgot to pick her up from the school bus stop like I would routinely do. I was under a lot of stress because their (her) brother was incarcerated with mental illness, and I would have trouble holding up emotionally depending upon the nature of the situation with him. She walked all the way from historic Auburn Ave to Freedom Parkway, where I worked. When I remembered to pick her up, I dashed out the door to discover she was not there and panicked, then called back to the office to hear from my co-worker that she had arrived there on foot.

I felt guilty and anxious about this mistake and can't remember, but I hoped my apology and time would heal her. Now, this is not to say that disappointments and a broken heart can bring about mental illness. But emotional pain can send a person down spiraling, which she later on did. She went on to high school, keeping up her grades, hanging with friends, and participating in extracurricular activities. Her Senior High School years would be more of the rezoning of students who would come from environments where fighting was survival. Later she would explain how miserable she was because of this, but in spite of this, she remained focused, joining the dance team marching band and won 2nd attendant school queen.

We gave her a lovely reception inviting family and friends after her high school graduation, which seemed to make her happy continuing to deal with more of the same (mental illness with her sib- lings). Plans for her to get accepted in an HBCU (Historical Black College University) were underway, as a freshman, her escape into her new world allowed her a level of freedom from the dismal life at home. She struggled her freshman year of college; now, here comes memories of all the situations and setbacks her siblings were having coming to haunt her making her college journey more complicated. She told me something that I completely forgot, and that was how she broke down emotionally. She fell completely apart and ended up in the college counselors' office as a result of her emotional state after telling them about her mentally unstable siblings and what she saw them going through.

The Counselor's next step was suggesting she had a diagnosis and to take medication which she completely denied. Keep in mind that her early years of trials were mixed up in a lot of disappointments and unexplained behaviors concerning her older siblings. She was blindsided by the fact that she had lost her identity, trying to figure out who she was behind the mental illness syndrome we were encountering all the time. Did this impact her emotionally? Yes, considering all that that she endured over the years. Taking matters into her own hands concerning her life, education, and what to do next, we saw her prioritizing go to another level and would not go well. She would end up in a physical altercation with a friend, almost jeopardizing her college career. One day, she explained. It started in the campus cafeteria, where she got into a verbal dispute with this friend and was not aware that the friend had a weapon, not to mention being pregnant. Wrong intentions to harm daughter#3 could have ended very badly as she verbally fought to defend herself, but by the Grace of God, didn't. This landed her before the School Board with consequences like community service and causing her to fail in her GPA.

I remember having to deal with this with her and seeing her in a state of fear, sadness, and regret. The community service mandate, however, turned into a light at the end of her tunnel. She had the opportunity to use her skilled training in Media Technology, putting together beautiful newsletters for the nonprofit community ministry. After all of this, her sophomore year, if I have it right, took a turn when she got her priorities in order and got serious about her studies, but she became pregnant before graduating from college. She didn't let that stop her and stunned us with her senior year accomplishments walking across the stage Cum Laude Graduation Day. Same as her 2nd older sibling, we were amazed and so very proud of her accomplishments. She was excited about her future, at least she appeared to be, and so were we. So, we were under the impression that returning to the city someday was inevitable for her, until one day, she announced that she would not be moving back, and she hasn't to this day. Blindsided this surprise as well as becoming grandparents, left us with feelings of mixed emotions. This new normal we were not ready to adjust to would change our world. I disappointed her by not showing up when she delivered my first grand-son, but our grandson's other grandparent did. Why? Most of us parents place an expectation on our children. I wanted my daughter to be married when she left home. I took for granted that once she left, she would not return. It was hard to explain to her that she couldn't return home because my marriage was strained, and I was headed into a collision with separation then divorce. This was harsh and put a barrier between our relationship for a long time.

We both suppressed feelings and con- tinued to keep supporting one another like families do. Never discussing in-depth a solution to all this, only made us all very uncomfortable emotionally. Sometime after that, she decided she would join the military to secure her and the new baby's future. Later on, we stepped in and took care of our grandson while she was away in military basic training which was very hard on her. I remember her calling home choked up with tears, explaining how they were treating her and saying harsh words and profane language. I explained to her that she belonged to the government now and was not sure what else was said, but words of encouragement were given to her, as always, I'm certain because that's what we did.

As our toddler grandson grew, we helped her as much as possible because we loved them both. Eventually, she married her baby's dad, and we gained another son-in-law. After she finished that training and returned home, I noticed she would change her hairstyles, going from thick lengthy hair to cutting it off (Big Chop); I heard it called. I thought to myself, maybe she's just tired of doing her hair, which many women tend to do. She decided she wanted to learn how to work on radio equipment with more training needed. Her ability to fix electrical things was unique. It noticeably seemed easy for her to do, which she seemed to enjoy. She returned home after completing this training, and we went out to dinner to celebrate her; while waiting to eat, I recall her blurting out, "mom, I think I have_____," immediately I went into denial and turned a deaf ear and don't even remember what else she said after that. In my state of shock, I told the devil-" you won't have this one," but still, I felt completely helpless again and very bad for her. I had to face reality and dealt with what I was about to take on again. This time with her being a new mommy and still wanting to be free to do what she wanted, we dealt with a lot of driving back and forth for an hour and a half down I-75 South to visit. I had been trained already with NAMI to handle these types of situations, but this was really tough because she lived a great distance from me, so this made me anxious and worried whether she was okay.

    She displayed such maturity growing up, captivating family members and her friends understanding how fam- ily life should be. Articulating it put her above her age group because she was so vocal about her way of seeing things, and expressing those thoughts clearly was one of her strong points. No one detected that she would be having her own personal inner struggles. I discovered her distancing herself from it all was her way of coping and never realizing she was suffering in silence. Perhaps these changes were part of what it would take for us to stay together. An old cliché that says, "absence makes the heart grow fonder", is true. However, I miss seeing her and her family because they live in another city. Desiring to help her in every way possible has been ongoing and worth it all. In fact, helping all 4 of my adult children and grandchildren has been worth its weight in gold, as strange as this may sound. My response and thoughts when her husband moved them three and a half hours away bothered me. She, being the youngest, took a leap of faith, allowing her to live her life the way she wanted felt strange. But we had to let go. This is a question for my readers as well CIT Crisis Intervention Team I like to ask when engaging the audience "if you saw your older siblings mentally sick after looking up to them, what would you do"? Some of the responses are " try to help them", or "think she may end up like her siblings with mental illness".

Instead, moving away from a toxic environment and family turned out to be her best solution. God only knows what she has endured watching all this mental sickness with her older siblings. It's taken courage on her part to seek professional help, to try to sort things within her soul. She is still a work in progress even through the trials of miscarrying their second child, in addition to their marriage ending. All this sent her down, spiraling and shattering her world.

It has taken much work on her part to help herself and hold her life together. By the Grace of God, they became pregnant again. Right after that birth a beautiful baby girl, she calls the "Rainbow Child", was born. It reminds you of God's promise made to Noah in the Bible after the Ark landed on dry land to look for the bow in the sky (Gen 9;13). The Lord keeps His promise; for that I'm grateful.

Our 3rd daughter and 4th child have managed to do such amazing work, from volunteering her time in the local community church, working full time in the job market, and now an entrepreneur (hair stylist) that has launched her business to a new level. She has put her business skills and hair craft technique into teaching classes to interested people how she creates braiding and innovative twists, etc., and distributes feminine women products. She loves social media and spending time with her family doing paint art projects as her therapy, she calls it, and all sorts of fun things with her two kids. She is still taking care of herself and has a good relationship with the children's dad.

Isa 6:13 second part of this verse says, "He will give a crown of beauty for ashes, a joyous blessing instead of mourning, festive praise instead of despair.

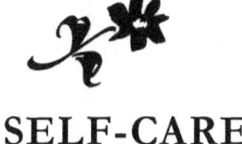

SELF-CARE

Blame Ourselves (NAMI Family Perspective)

As a result of confrontations and irregularities in my life because of the mental illness I blamed myself, I became fussy, irritable, and very impatient. I've failed quite a bit but come to realize that everything happening to us with this mental illness disease and anything else that came with it was not all my fault. Every time there has been a crisis with my children and their illness, it has set me back, never getting the breath to push or lunge forward. I want to run in the opposite direction but, in my heart, I know I can't. I learned through trials and tribulations to stand on God's word and that it had to become first in my life. Suffering with anxiety symptoms, not knowing to call it that early on caused me to talk fast and walk fast most of my adult life, hurriedly running into a brick wall eventually. I was desperate as a mother, desiring to seek help for her children. What came out of this not attending to myself were palpitations (racing heartbeat). One day, while working at my place of employment in the Atlanta Public School System, which I'm a product of, I had a panic attack. I began to freak out, thinking that this was it. I have pushed myself to the point that now I'm getting sick. I phoned the paramedics and asked them if they would park out of sight because I didn't want my boss to see me slip out to see them. After they arrived, I shared what I was dealing with and that it had been ongoing for quite some time. One of the paramedics began to chuckle, then remarked that I had residuals leftover from dealing with so much of this stuff (mental illness). They advised me to see a doctor and get counseling because I had suppressed so many crisis episodes. I didn't coin the phrase "it's tight, but it's right", and I had been in a tight place dealing with mental illness from day one. I slipped back into work, and my boss saw me and shouted my name anxiously, asking if I was okay.

I explained to her what was happening to me and tried to deal with it without bringing attention to myself. She understood and encouraged me to do what I needed to take care of myself. There are no quick fixes or answers, and this roller coaster ride handicapped my ability to function. I wanted to get off of it, so I sought professional help along with prayer, and by the grace of God, my process began. A friend recommended a christian counselor who would open with prayer before listening to me. Many other challenges I've faced since then, over the course of time, the Lord took over (where I left off). After I moved out of the way, I turned it over to the Lord and began to listen to the Holy Spirit's instructions more. The Lord had me move further south so that I could attend NAMI Family Support Group at a church in the community. I'm so grateful that I was able to finish this Book Project in God's timing.

Here are some things I do for Self-Care:

- Attend NAMI Family Support Group Meetings
- Counseling(individual)

- Go to a Movie (and get a good belly laugh)
- Massage(30min) once a month
- Bible Study with women's group
- Walking Trail (30 min) with a friend
- Pray daily (which is first and foremost)

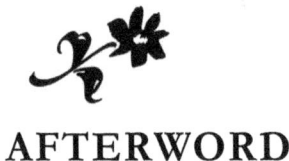

AFTERWORD

At the end of each chapter, I was led to quote a scripture over our adult children's lives to empower them and hope family members will follow this model by doing the same. It's easy to say the wrong words when we are frustrated, angry, or even sad- but try; it will push you forward.

God has set a platform for me to train with Law Enforcement as an advocate and NAMI family member, which was my way of serving and giving back to the mental health community, movement and system. Today, I've learned that I have to face and deal with my issues in life. It was a motivational speaker that quoted something like this, "Do I deal with it gracefully, you are probably asking, and my answer is NO". But for the grace of GOD and the support of a network of family members and community, we have strengthened ourselves.

If an ill family member is taken to ER and held 24 to 72 hours, it's vital that the family get the loved one to a CSB (Community Service Board) or a BH (Behavioral Health Center) to stabilize them. Don't allow yourselves to shut down and not communicate because of fear that your sick family member may be hostile. Ask the tough questions "do you need a prescription filled" when they show signs such as (not eating, bathing regularly, isolation, looking depressed, or the silent treatment).

Often these loved ones need medication refills. Remember, don't overreact and be suspicious of them. They like their privacy but, you have to check in with them, see if they need anything. Get in touch with your local NAMI support group, join and become a member of this movement and talk it out. Don't focus on conversations about your loved ones with the illness; but exchange strength in sharing your own personal experiences, resources. Talk about how you, as the "Over Comer" and family member, have beat this disease called mental illness. Get training through NAMI on as much information as possible about the brain's function and medications. Become involved in your local State level NAMI Support Movement, attend the annual National Convention, and join to learn more.

Mental illness is a harsh reality. Even for some of us when matters occur that put us in a state of losing self-control is also a reality. Mental illness may or may not ever go away. But I have heard testimonies and seen individual's struggles; how they were healed, delivered, and set free of this illness. It depends on the individual because we were each created differently. We have to take our heads out of the sand, pull ourselves up by our bootstraps and dig in reading up on medical terms, study how the brain functions when mental illness strikes. "We never give up hope" is one of the Principles of support from the Family support Meeting Group model of NAMI. Here's a list of all of the Principle of Support:

1. We will see the individual first, not the illness
2. We recognize that mental illnesses are medical illnesses that may

have environmental triggers

3. We understand that mental illnesses are traumatic events

4. We aim for better coping skills

5. We find strength in sharing experiences

6. We reject stigma in ourselves and others

7. We won't judge anyone's pain as less than our own

8. We forgive ourselves and reject guilt

9. We embrace humor as healthy

10. We accept we cannot resolve all problems

11. We expect a better future in a realistic way

12. We never give up hope

I have overcome the shame, blame, and guilt syndrome. I work hard at letting others know that there is hope and a cure. Psalm 139 God, says, as I paraphrase His ways are not our ways, His thoughts are not our thoughts, they are too deep and wonderful". I finally came to the conclusion to look to God and stop doing it my way. I thought it would work because "Recovery Is Good Business" we march on personally and help others stay on the road to recovery.

There are 4 Points I want to leave with you taken from Dr. Lloyd Sederer YouTube X Ted Talks:

- DON'T GO IT ALONE
- DON'T GET INTO FIGHTS
- LEARN THE MENTAL HEALTH SYSTEM
- It's A MARATHON NOT A SPRINT

RESOURCES

NAMI (National Alliance on Mental Illness) 1-888-999-6264 for NAMI Georgia-770-234-0855 or your Local State NAMI Office.

BHL (Behavioral Health Link) Georgia Crisis & Access Line 1-800-715-4225),

GMHCN (Georgia Mental Health Consumer Network) 1-800-297-6146,

Local CSB (Community Service Board), County Shelters, Group Homes, Non-Profit Organizations that aid families with mental illness. County Subsidized Housing Programs/Supportive Employment.

DBHDD (Department Behavioral Health & Development) 404-657-2252, GCSA (Georgia Council on Substance Abuse) 1-844-325-5400. NSPL (National Suicide Prevention Lifeline) 1-800-273-8255

Note: here is the link (www.chaplaindelora.com) for my blog and social media website page for you to share, ask questions, and give your experience of how you're coping with a family with mental illness. I will reply with as many resources along with encouraging words as possible to help you get through your process.

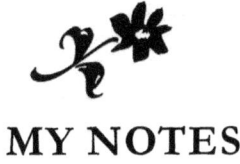
MY NOTES

My Notes

My Notes

My Notes

My Notes

My Notes

My Notes

My Notes

www.ingramcontent.com/pod-product-compliance
Lightning Source LLC
Chambersburg PA
CBHW030302030426
42336CB00009B/484